Protect Against Diabetes

Learn The Secret Of Berries And Spice (Without Drugs, Type I & II, Treatment, Overcome, Prevent)

Sherry S. Williams

Protect Against Diabetes: Learn The Secret Of Berries And Spice (Without Drugs, Type I & II, Treatment, Overcome, Prevent)

This book was self-published with the amazing help of Self-Publishing Made Easy Now! [1] . You can grab a free copy of the checklist that started my journey here: FREE Self-Publishing Checklist [2] .

[1] https://selfpublishingmadeeasynow.com/xpjv

[2] https://selfpublishingmadeeasynow.com/free_checklist

Table of Contents

Chapter 1 – Introduction

Diabetes mellitus, simply known as diabetes, is now the fastest growing health concern throughout the world. The disease is a result of a malfunction of the body's production and utilization of insulin. It is a serious problem considered as an epidemic.

In the US alone, around 17 million or 6.2 percent of the country's population suffers from the disease but about 5.9 million of them aren't even aware that they already have it. It was estimated by the World Health Organization (WHO) that by the year 2025, about 300 million people from around the world will have diabetes.

Insulin is important because the body uses it in converting food, starches, and sugar into energy. When you have diabetes, your body cannot use blood sugar or glucose for energy. As a result, your blood glucose levels will rise and you will suffer from hyperglycemia. When this happens, your body will get rid of sugar through urination. In worst cases, it is possible for a diabetic person to end up starving to death.

2 - Three Types of Diabetes

The following are the three main types of diabetes:

Type 1

This used to be called juvenile diabetes but is now more commonly referred to as insulin-dependent since it is treated using insulin. It usually affects young adults and children. It happens when the pancreas malfunctions and stops from producing sufficient amounts of insulin.

Type 2

This is also referred to as adult-onset diabetes or noninsulin dependent because it is linked to insulin resistant cells. Older adults are more at risk of developing this kind of disease, but it is now also found in younger individuals, such as children and teens.

Gestational or pregnancy-related

There are certain women who develop the disease during and until the end of their pregnancy. It typically goes away after they have given birth, but it puts them at a higher risk of developing Type 2 diabetes later in life.

3 - The Symptoms

The symptoms of this disease develop gradually. More often than not, people don't recognize that they are experiencing the symptoms so they remain unaware that they have it.

Here are some of the symptoms, which indicate that you may already be suffering from diabetes:

- Poor sleeping habits

- Extreme thirst and hunger

- Sudden weight loss

- Frequent urination

- Feeling tired all the time

- Infections and wounds that take longer to heal

- Tingling sensation or numbness in the hands and feet

- Very dry skin

There are some people who suffer from two or more of these symptoms, but there are also those who don't experience any of them. However, if you want to be certain, it is always best to speak to your doctor and get tested.

4 - Unhealthy Lifestyle Leads to Diabetes

The alarming rise of diabetes in recent years is attributed to these two unhealthy lifestyle habits – poor diet and lack of exercise.

An average person these days consumes twice the protein and calories than what is required. People eat a lot of the bad stuff – simple sugars, pasta, French fries, candies, ice cream, etc. It is okay to eat these foods but only in moderation. The problem is that you take in more than 160 pounds of sugars and sweeteners in a year that your body does not need at all.

Just imagine what would happen when your body takes in more unhealthy food and you don't exercise enough but instead, smoke and drink alcohol frequently. All these unhealthy habits lead to stress, weight gain, and diseases that include diabetes.

If you have any of the following signs, you better have yourself checked so that you can get treated before the disease becomes worse:

4 - UNHEALTHY LIFESTYLE LEADS TO DIABETES

- You are physically inactive.

- You are more than 20 percent overweight.

- You have a history of gestational diabetes or you have given birth to a baby that weighed 9 pounds and above.

- You have a family history of diabetes.

- Your triglycerides levels are above 250 milligrams per deciliter.

- Your HDL cholesterol or good cholesterol is below 35 milligrams per deciliter.

- You have a history of high blood pressure and hypertension.

- Your previous blood tests indicated that you have Impaired Glucose Tolerance (IGF) or Impaired Fasting Glucose (IFG).

5 - The Right Herbs and Spices for Preventing Diabetes

It is necessary to maintain your sugar levels at a normal rate to protect yourself from diabetes and improve your overall health. You can do this by following a healthy diet, having a regular exercise routine, staying away from vices, and having a regular check-up with your doctor.

There are many things that you can do to control your blood sugar levels without spending a lot. Here's a list of herbs and spices that can help in protecting you against diabetes:

Cinnamon

Cinnamon is considered as one of the oldest spices. It comes from the brown bark of the cinnamon tree. The bark is dried before it is turned into either a cinnamon stick or ground powder.

This spice has bioactive components that act as an insulin substitute if you have type 2 of diabetes. It also has a positive effect on a person's triglyceride levels, HDL cholesterol, LDL cholesterol, and fasting plasma glucose. It has the ability to triple the efficiency of your insulin. It is important to take note that you cannot take this spice if you are taking any kinds of blood-thinning medication.

How do you take this spice? You can take it in the form of supplements. Make sure that you consult your doctor for the right dosage suitable for your overall health. You can also add a dash or two of the spice to your smoothies, oatmeal, pastries, and dishes. You can also take up to 2 grams of cinnamon tea every day.

Turmeric

This spice is more known as the ingredient that gives curry its distinct yellow color. Turmeric contains curcumin, a compound rich in medicinal benefits that include the prevention of diabetes by controlling your blood sugar levels. It has other health benefits due to its anti-atherosclerotic, anti-inflammatory, weight-reducing, heart-protecting, and antioxidant properties.

There are studies, which proved that taking a daily dose of 1.5 grams of curcumin for 9 months leads to the prevention of having type 2 diabetes. According to these studies, the component curcumin helped in improving a person's beta-cell function. It also plays an important role in preventing kidney-related complications for diabetic people.

You can take turmeric as a supplement but ask your doctor for the right dosage. Generally, you can include powdered or raw turmeric in various dishes to benefit from its health benefits.

Black Curry or Black Seed

Black curry is scientifically known as Nigella sativa. It comes from a flower's seed that has been used for medicinal purposes since the ancient times. It has a lot of health benefits that include lower blood pressure, effective acne control, asthma relief, reduce joint pain, stronger immune system, and fight against the superbugs.

This spice that adds a pungent bitter flavor to foods has a powerful anti-diabetic activity. It helps in preventing possible complications that may arise from having diabetes. It controls your blood sugar levels and reduces your fasting blood sugar. It also lowers the levels of your blood lipids.

Black seed oil is commonly used in the prevention of diabetes. A study in 2015 found out that the seeds contain dietary components that maintain the proper levels of fats and glucose in the blood. The oil helps in the restoration of the normal levels of glucose, reduces oxidative stress, and improves sensitivity to insulin.

It prevents cardiovascular problems that may arise due to diabetes. Aside from prevention, the seeds can help in treating the disease by taking them in pill form at a dose of 2 grams every day along with your other medicines.

Ginger

This spice, popularly used as an ingredient in many dishes, is also known for its medicinal benefits that include the prevention and improvement of diabetes symptoms. It has antioxidant and anti-inflammatory properties that make your heart and eyes healthier. It also has anti-oxidative, hypolipidemic, and anti-diabetic properties. It can also improve cholesterol levels, reduce oxidative stress, and boost insulin sensitivity.

Taking 2 to 3 grams of ginger on a daily basis can help in reducing your fasting blood sugar and in regulating your blood sugar levels. According to a 2014 study, a patient with Type 2 diabetes can benefit from 3 capsules (1-gram) of ginger powder for two months.

Ginger is beneficial to your overall health and can even aid in the weight loss process. You can add fresh or dried ginger to your dishes. You can also make ginger tea and take up to 3 cups a day.

Fenugreek

This herb regulates your blood sugar levels and decreases your fasting blood sugar. It helps in improving your glucose tolerance due to its hypoglycemic activity. You can reduce your risk of developing diabetes by taking fenugreek regularly for 3 years. Soak up to 2 tablespoons of the seeds in water overnight. You can eat the seeds and drink the water the following day. You can also benefit from its positive health effects by using fenugreek flour in baking goods.

Onion

Onion is a delicious spice used in many dishes. It also has many health benefits due to its active hypoglycemic substances. Aside from preventing diabetes, eating 100 grams of raw red onion can help those who are already suffering from the disease by lowering their blood sugar levels. It is easy to take since you can add it to your food.

Coriander

Coriander, also called cilantro has lipid-lowering and anti-oxidant effects. Its extracts help in breaking down complex carbohydrates into sugars.

Banaba Leaf

This plant, which is native to Southeast Asia, India, and the Philippines, is known for its medicinal properties. It is usually brewed into a tea and taken directly without any sugar added. The tea helps in preventing diabetes and it also aids in the weight loss process. Banaba extracts help in inducing the transport of glucose to the body cells through the blood. The leaf of the plant contains an active ingredient known as corosolic acid, responsible for regulating the blood sugar levels.

Momordica Charantia

This plant is commonly called bitter melon or bitter gourd, an apt name since all parts of the plant is bitter. It helps regulate blood sugar levels and has other medicinal purposes and benefits. It is used in treating fever, intestinal worm, dysentery, and colitis. It helps in preventing diabetes with its anti-diabetic properties – polypeptide-p, vicine, and charantin.

It contains lectin, responsible for reducing blood glucose. It is loaded with iron, vitamins C, B1, B2, and A. Regular intake of bitter melon prevents complications usually experienced by diabetics, such as neuritis, eye problems, and difficulty in the metabolism of carbs.

Garlic

Garlic is good for cardiovascular health and can also help in preventing diabetes. It helps fight inflammation and lowers the blood sugar levels due to its hypolipidemic and anti-diabetic properties. It has sulfur compounds that maintain healthy cholesterol levels and protect against oxidative stress.

To benefit from its health benefits, make it a habit to add garlic to your dishes. You can also eat up to 3 raw garlic cloves on an empty stomach every day.

Aloe Vera

This medicinal plant has various uses and it is now available as an oral supplement that can help improve diabetes symptoms. It is effective in reducing fasting blood sugar and in maintaining healthy levels of blood sugar. It also benefits your overall health due to the presence of its compounds, such as anthraquinones, mannans, and lectins.

Taking aloe vera juice can help improve your blood sugar levels. It helps in healing wounds faster and in decreasing the lipids or fats in the blood.

Jambu fruit

Jamboline is found in its seed, which prevents the conversion of too much starch into sugar. The seed in powdered form can be added to buttermilk or water to reduce the amount of sugar in urine.

Curry Patta

Make it a habit to eat 10 fresh leaves in the morning for 12 weeks to keep yourself diabetes-free.

Bael Leaves

You can make fresh juice from the leaves and add a dash of pepper for a refreshing and anti-diabetic beverage.

Curry Leaves

Curry leaf powder has hypoglycemic properties that control postprandial and fasting blood glucose levels. The leaves contain minerals that help in maintaining healthy levels of blood sugar, prevent oxidative stress, and boost the body's metabolism of carbohydrates.

In order to prevent diabetes, you can make it a habit to add curry leaf powder to your salads, dishes, and soups. You can also chew some tender curry leaves first thing in the morning on an empty stomach.

6 - Berries and Other Superfoods for Diabetes Prevention

Berries are good for our general health but they are also considered to be an essential part of a diabetic diet. Berries are low in glycemic index. Foods with high GI or the types that score higher than 70 tend to raise blood sugar levels. The opposite happens when you take in foods with low GI score. Berries, such as raspberries, blackberries, blueberries, and strawberries score below 40.

Berries are loaded with polyphenols, which include anthocyanins, and potent anti-oxidant properties. These properties make berries ideal not only in preventing diabetes, but also in enhancing brain functions, weight loss, anti-cancer, anti- arteriosclerosis, and in improving vascular and visual activities.

Here are the kinds of berries that can help in preventing diabetes:

Blueberries

Blueberries are loaded with phytonutrients, chemicals derived from plants that offer lots of health benefits. They include resveratrol, flavonols, hydroxybenzoic acids, hydroxy-cinnamic acids, and anthocyanins. They give the fruits their anti-inflammatory and antioxidant properties.

By consuming up to 2 cups of blueberries per day, your good cholesterol (HDL) will increase, and the bad cholesterol (LDL) and triglycerides will decrease. The fruit is also effective in maintaining a healthy blood pressure. Its anti-oxidant properties protect your nerve cells from damage caused by oxidative stress. The juice and fruit of a blueberry enhance a person's memory and slow down the decline of the brain functions.

Blueberries will not cause any spike in your blood sugar level because of their low GI score. People who have type 2 diabetes usually eat 3 servings of the fruit to improve their blood sugar levels. You can take these berries along with other fruits with low GI scores. These berries are loaded with fiber, soluble and insoluble. Soluble fiber helps im-prove your blood sugar control. Insoluble fiber gets rid of the fat in your system.

Aside from diabetes prevention, these berries have vitamins A and C, antioxidants, and folate, which help in fighting off cancer cells and in slowing down the progress of the disease. A serving of blueberries or half a cup gives off zero grams of fat, 2 grams of fiber, 11 grams of carbohydrate, and 42 calories.

You can enjoy the fruit as it is or you can add it to your morning meals and cereals, or as an added flavor to your salad or yogurt. It has been found out that taking about 2 1/2 cups of wild blueberry juice each day for 3 months is effective in lowering blood glucose levels and in making you feel better.

Strawberries

This is said to be the most popular berry in the United States but is found in many parts of the world. This is a favorite ingredient in many dishes, pastries, and desserts. Similar to blueberries, strawberries are also rich in antioxidants.

A daily serving of 2 cups of strawberries per day is effective in lowering your LDL cholesterol and in reducing the risk of women from suffering from a stroke. These berries are rich in potassium, which is an effective element in lowering a person's blood pressure. They also have antioxidant properties that prevent the formation of blood clots.

Strawberries have a low GI score, which makes them ideal for a diabetic diet. Having around 3 servings of strawberries per week can decrease your chances of developing Type 2 of diabetes. There are studies, which proved that eating around 37 pieces of the fruit can lower your risk of diabetes complications, such as neuropathy and kidney disease. You can also eat the fruit with a bit of table sugar to reduce the spike of blood glucose that you can get from the table sugar.

Similar to blueberries, strawberries are also used in blocking the growth of tumors in cancer by decreasing the inflammation. From a serving of one cup of fresh berries, you will get zero grams of fat, 3 grams of fiber, 11 grams of carbohydrate, and 46 calories. This fruit is versatile. You can turn it into a smoothie or use as flavor to your dishes, dips, and salsa.

The other berries that are ideal for a diabetic diet include blackberries and raspberries. They contain low carbohydrates, low GI scores, and loaded with essential vitamins and nutrients necessary in preventing the disease.

Other Anti-Diabetes Superfoods

Aside from berries, herbs, and spices, here's a list of foods considered as superfoods in diabetes prevention and cure:

Broccoli

This vegetable has sulforaphane, a compound that triggers anti-inflammatory effects that protect blood vessels and improve blood sugar levels. It protects the heart from the damages that may arise as a result of the disease. The compound also activates the natural detox mechanism of the body that protects the system against other diseases, including cancer.

Dark chocolate

It is loaded with flavonoids that decrease fasting blood glucose and insulin levels, boost insulin sensitivity, reduce insulin resistance and suppress appetite. Dark chocolate is also good for the heart because it lowers your risk of a stroke, heart attack, and high blood pressure.

Olive oil

It contains monounsaturated fats and antioxidant properties that protect the body against diabetes and other diseases, such as heart ailments.

Spinach

This vegetable is rich in vitamin K and minerals, such as zinc, folate, phosphorous, magnesium, and potassium. It is recommended to eat more than one serving of this veggie or combine it with other leafy greens to reduce your risk of diabetes by 14 percent.

Steel-cut oats

The amount of magnesium in these oats helps your system in secreting insulin and in using glucose properly. Whole grains are rich in fiber, antioxidants, and nutrients. Studies have found out that a diet rich in magnesium, and whole grains are effective in lowering a person's risk of developing Type 2 diabetes.

Walnuts

The nuts that come from the most prevalent tree nut in the world, are rich in alpha-linolenic acid, a polyunsaturated fatty acid effective in lowering inflammation. This food is good for general health due to its anti-high cholesterol, anti-viral, anticancer, and antioxidant properties. These characteristics of walnuts are essential in reversing the progress of heart ailments and diabetes.

Thank You

As we reach the end of this book, I want to say thanks for reading this book.

I want to get this information out to as many people as possible. If you found this book helpful, I would greatly appreciate you leaving me a review. This helps others find the book as well.

This book was self-published with the amazing help of <u>Self-Publishing Made Easy Now!</u> [3] . You can grab a free copy of the checklist that started my journey here: <u>FREE Self-Publishing Checklist</u> [4] .

[3] https://selfpublishingmadeeasynow.com/xpjv
[4] https://selfpublishingmadeeasynow.com/free_checklist

Disclaimer

This document is geared towards providing exact and reliable information in regards to the topic and issue covered. The publication is sold on the idea that the publisher is not required to render an accounting, officially permitted, or otherwise, qualified services. If advice is necessary, legal, financial, medical or professional, a practiced individual in the profession should be ordered.

This information is not presented by a financial or medical practitioner and is for entertainment, educational and informational purposes only. The content is not intended as a substitute for professional medical advice, diagnosis, or treatment.

Always seek the advice of your physician or other qualified health care provider with any questions you may have regarding a medical condition. Never disregard professional medical advice or delay in seeking it because of something you have read.

The information provided herein is stated to be truthful and consistent, in that any liability, in terms of inattention or otherwise, by any usage or abuse of any policies, processes, or directions contained within is the solitary and utter re-

DISCLAIMER

sponsibility of the recipient reader.

Under no circumstances will any legal responsibility or blame be held against the publisher for any reparation, damages, or monetary loss due to the information herein, either directly or indirectly.